ANTI-INFLAMMATORY DIET

The Ultimate Cookbook With

Easy and Tasty Recipes

Dakota Boyer

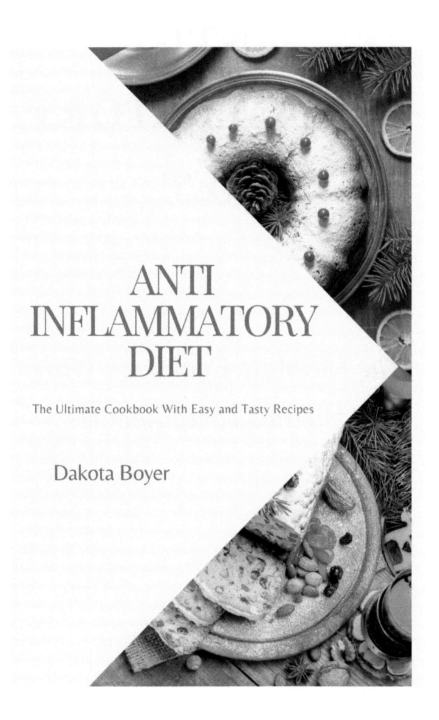

ANTI INFLAMMATORY DIET

The Ultimate Cookbook With Easy and Tasty Recipes

Dakota Boyer

Table of Contents

The following Book is reproduced below with the goal of providing information that is as accurate and reliable as possible. Regardless, purchasing this Book can be seen as consent to the fact that both the publisher and the author of this book are in no way experts on the topics discussed within and that any recommendations or suggestions that are made herein are for entertainment purposes only. Professionals should be consulted as needed prior to undertaking any of the action endorsed herein.
This declaration is deemed fair and valid by both the American Bar Association and the Committee of Publishers Association and is legally binding throughout the United States.

The information in the following pages is broadly considered a truthful and accurate account of facts and as such, any inattention, use, or misuse of the information in question by the reader will render any resulting actions solely under their purview. There are no scenarios in which the publisher or the original author of this work can be in any fashion deemed liable for any hardship or damages that may befall them after undertaking information described herein.

Additionally, the information in the following pages is intended only for informational purposes and should thus be thought of as universal. As befitting its nature, it is presented without assurance regarding its prolonged validity or interim quality. Trademarks that are mentioned are done without written consent and can in no way be considered an endorsement from the trademark holder.

INTRODUCTION

Regardless of your awareness, inflammation naturally happens to you as an essential part of your body's immunity system. It is a beneficial process because it protects our body from dangerous invaders such as bacteria and viruses. At the same time, inflammation is a significant factor in developing chronic diseases, precisely because you may not even know that it is happening most of the time. Besides medications and drugs, there are ways you can fight inflammations naturally and even prevent unpleasant health issues and chronic disease. The best part is that, fortunately, you have complete control over it through your diet.

I struggled for years with acne, bloated belly, irregular periods, and unexplained fatigue. Then I discovered that all these medical conditions resulted from inflammation in my gut, and since I started to control what I eat, my body and my whole-being had massive improvements. From time to time, I like to remind myself that every particle within my body is made of what I eat.

You cannot underestimate the importance of your daily nutritional intake and the quality of the food that you consume. Especially today that, unless you look for organic and raw produce, you must read every single food label carefully. Pesticides, additives, toxins, and even particles of plastic are hidden in your food.

It is easy to understand how certain foods can trigger your inflammatory response that weakens your body, preventing it from functioning at its best. Keto may be controversial, but health benefits for a wide range of various health conditions have now been reported and documented. Keto naturally reduces inflammatory foods, but following a keto diet does not necessarily mean that you are eating healthier and properly fighting inflammation.

A ketogenic diet has some anti-inflammatory benefits, but focusing on fat and eliminating entire categories of foods is not a wise way to achieve radiant well-being. Therefore, some people experience inflammation while on a keto. Others focus too much on process keto-friendly food rather than making and cooking whole, fresh, and minimal process food a priority. People who tend to focus more on ketones are also the ones who struggle to achieve their health goals.
To enhance the best food-as-medicine from your keto diet and optimizing what you eat upon your goals is essential to achieve good results. You can replace particular keto food with alternative anti-inflammatory keto-friendly products in your diet to lower inflammation, with no guilt. However, it is crucial to understand that it is not only about dieting and following a meal plan but also about establishing good habits, providing optimal nutrition to our body, and developing a healthier lifestyle.

As I am susceptible to people with particular health conditions, I would like to emphasize a couple of points before continuing.

- Take the nutritional information reported in the recipes as a guideline, and they can vary to a great extent from brand to brand. They have been calculated by using online nutritional calculators, which do not guarantee accuracy.
- This anti-inflammatory cookbook kick start is not one-size-fits-all. Please speak with your dietitian or nutritionist before starting the plan to determine your caloric needs.

A ketogenic diet done well can have an enormous impact on your well-being, improving your longevity and health.

EATING KETO TO LOWER INFLAMMATION

Keto may be controversial, but people that 'are gone keto' report health benefits for a wide range of various health conditions: heart disease, cancer, Alzheimer, epilepsy, brain injuries, and Parkinson. Keto can also help with diabetes, predicates from different points of view, and it is a very efficient way to lose weight.

The main benefits of ketogenic diets:

RAPID WEIGHT LOSS: Low-carb diets drastically reduce your appetite, and consequently, cutting cubs, you end up eating more proteins and fewer calories. However, low-carb diets seem to have an effect only on short-terms.

TRIGLYCERIDES DROP: Eating carbs is one of the main reasons why triglycerides increase in sedentary people. Low-carb diets reduce the fat molecules in the bloodstream reducing the risk of heart disease.

LOW BLOOD PRESSURE: Reducing blood pressure means lowering the risk of common diseases as well.

BALANCE CHOLESTEROL: Low-carb diets include a lot of good fat, which is responsible for increasing HDL levels, lowering the risk of heart diseases. At the same time, it also increases the size of LDL particles reducing their harmful effect.

REDUCE BLOOD SUGAR AND INSULIN: The best way to reduce blood sugar and insulin levels is by cutting carbs. In one study, people with diabetes reduced the insulin intake by 50% when they started a low-carb diet.

BETTER GUMS: Gum diseases and toothaches are commonly caused by the consumption of too much sugar. Even so, following a keto diet does not necessarily mean that you are eating healthier, regardless of its version (Standard, cyclical, targeted, or high proteins ketogenic diet (*)). One of the disadvantages that keto can cause is some sort of disorder within your digestive system, provoking diarrhea, bloating, and other unpleasant symptoms. Therefore, some people experience inflammation while on a keto. Others focus too much on process keto- friendly food rather than making and cooking whole, fresh, and minimal process food a priority. People who tend to focus more on ketones (the metabolic state that your body uses to burn fat instead of fat) are also the ones who struggle to achieve their health goals. Keto naturally reduces most inflammatory foods, but, as in all the diets, particular foods are healthier than others. Optimizing what you eat upon your goals is essential to achieve good results.

To enhance the best food-as-medicine from your keto diet, replace particular keto food with alternative anti-inflammatory keto-friendly products. Some anti-inflammatory foods can be introduced with no guilt in your keto diet to lower inflammation. For example, swop all the processed keto bars, desserts, and shakes with homemade sugar-free fat bombs, nutty spreads, or any sugar and dairy-free keto treat.

A keto diet done well can also prevent chronic diseases, reduce pain from inflammation and, overall, improve your longevity and health. However, it is crucial to understand that it is not only about dieting and following a meal plan but also about establishing good habits, providing optimal nutrition to our body, and developing a healthier lifestyle.

(*) STANDARD (SKD): 70% fat – 20% protein – 10% carbs. **CYCLICAL (CKD):** 5 days of Standard keto diet followed by 2 high carbs days (designed for athletes and bodybuilders).

TARGETED (TKD): It allows adding carbs around workouts (designed for athletes and bodybuilders).

HIGH PROTEIN: 60% fat – 35% proteins – 5% carbs.

ANTI-INFLAMMATORY FRIENDLY FOOD

PROTEINS

Poultry: Free-range chicken, turkey, Cornish hen, quail, goose, pheasant, and duck.

Fish and Seafood: Salmon, cod, tuna, scrod, anchovies, mackerel, flounder, catfish, calamari, mahi-mahi, halibut, sole, sardines, halibut, snapper, sardines, and trout. Go for wild-caught fish to avoid toxins present in commercially raised fish.

Grass-Fed Meat: These include beef, goat, lamb, and venison, in moderation. Meat from wild animals is also acceptable; Choose the chunks of meat with more fat since they contain less protein and more fat.

Pork: Pork Loin and ham have antioxidative and anti-inflammatory effects; as a result, they decrease free radicals and reduce inflammation.

Whole Eggs: Eggs are one of the best anti-inflammatory foods thanks to their high content of vitamin D, which regulates the inflammatory response in rheumatoid arthritis. This includes chicken eggs and quail.

Shellfish: Oyster, clams, scallops, mussels, lobster, shrimps, crab (not imitation crab that contains additives), and squid. They are loaded with nutrients that may promote heart health, including omega-3 fatty acids and vitamin B12.

FATS AND OILS

Good fats are the main sauce of energy while on this diet. **Omega 3:** Fatty acids from shellfish and fatty fish like tuna and salmon. **Monounsaturated fats:** Such as avocado, egg yolks, and grass-fed butter. **Vegetable oils:** Such as extra-virgin coconut oil and extra-virgin olive oil.

FRESH VEGETABLES:

Unless you grow your own to avoid all pesticide toxins, opt for organic ones. Avoid starchy vegetables (corn, potatoes, peas, and winter squash) that are high in carbs. Control the intake of sweet vegetables (squashes, peppers, tomatoes, and carrots).

Research shows that vitamin K-rich leafy greens like spinach, kale, broccoli, and cabbage reduce inflammation.

Fresh vegetables that make it to the list are alfalfa sprouts, asparagus, bamboo shoots, bean sprouts, broccoli, brussels sprouts, celery, cabbage, cauliflower, celery root, chard, beet greens, bok choy, chives, collard greens, cucumbers, dandelion greens, dill pickles, garlic, green onions (high in sugar; moderate intake), kale, leeks, mushrooms, olives, radishes, salad greens, and lettuces (romaine, arugula, fennel, Boston lettuce, endive, Mache, escarole, sorrel, radicchio, chicory) water chestnuts, sauerkraut, scallions, shallots, shallots, snow peas, spinach, swiss chard, turnips...go for a variety of colors! **Spinach:** They holds plenty of antioxidants as well as many agents that relieve inflammation and help fight diseases.

Kale: This is a nutrient-dense, detoxifying food packed with anti- inflammatory properties. Kale contains various amino acids, vitamins A, C, and K, and a variety of antioxidants that prevent cellular damage.

Broccoli: They are another anti-inflammatory powerhouse. Rich in vitamins K and C, folate, fiber, and packed with antioxidants.

Cabbage: It contains many different antioxidants that reduce certain blood markers of inflammation and chronic inflammation.

FRESH FRUITS:

Most fruits and berries contain quite a lot of carbs; that is why they taste sweet.

Low-carb fruits that make it to the list are: Watermelon, raspberry, cantaloupe, star fruit, rhubarb, cherry, apple, lemon, and blueberry (in moderation).

Avocado is an extraordinary source of healthy monounsaturated fat and antioxidants.

Tomato is a nutritional powerhouse! Tomatoes have impressive anti- inflammatory properties and loaded with potassium and vitamin C. **Strawberry:** It has plenty of anti-inflammatory and antioxidant health benefits.

Peach: It is power-packed with antioxidants and has anti-inflammatory properties. Peaches are high in dietary fiber and bring along a surfeit of vitamins and minerals like vitamin A, C, E, and K, potassium, phosphorous, magnesium, calcium, and a bit of protein.

DAIRY PRODUCTS :

Dairy is a vast category. Generally speaking, fermented products, like yogurt and kefir, are anti-inflammatory, are welcome, whereas products high in saturated fat, such as cheeses and ice cream, may promote inflammation. Always opt for raw milk products, and if you do not have easy access to them, go for the organic labels.

Kefir: This is a great probiotic source as it contains anti-mycotic, anti- neoplastic, antibacterial, and immunomodulatory properties.

Yogurt: It presents proteins and probiotics with anti-inflammatory and immunomodulatory roles, and its daily consumption can prevent gut microbiota alteration. Plain Greek yogurt is the best option: healthier, higher protein content, and lower in carbs than other yogurts.

Feta: Feta cheese contains friendly bacteria that promote intestinal and immune intestinal health, in addition to their anti-inflammatory effects. **Mozzarella:** It also contains bacteria that act as probiotics improving gut health, promoting immunity, and fighting inflammation.

Goat: Goat cheese contains a unique fatty acid profile that has been associated with several health benefits. For example, dairy products made from goat's milk have been shown to possess anti-inflammatory properties and may even help decrease hunger.

Pecorino: It is not only delicious, but it has health benefits too. It is rich in calcium, potassium, and magnesium and is a good source of protein. It also contains high amounts of omega 3, which are beneficial in preventing cardiovascular diseases, improving immune function, reducing inflammation, improving vision and learning, and slowing down mental deterioration.

BEVERAGES :

Vegetable kinds of milk are not created equally. While some are incredibly nutritious and healthy, others have some drawbacks. Almonds, coconut, and hemp milk are the best options for an anti-inflammatory boost.

Coconut milk: It has anti-inflammatory and antibiotic benefits. It also may aid weight loss by lowering your appetite, balancing your microbiome and blood sugar levels.

Almond milk: It has an outstanding profile. It is rich in vitamin E and magnesium. Reduce bad cholesterol and lower triglycerides. Increase good cholesterol. Besides regulating your blood sugar levels, almond milk may also benefit your heart.

Cashew milk contains antioxidants. It helps to balance your blood sugar levels, and it may lower inflammation and boost your immune system. Hemp milk is a good source of healthy fats, protein, calcium, and iron. It is rich in Omega-3 fatty acids, reduces inflammation, protects your skin health, and reduces signs of aging.

Coffee: It contains antioxidants, and moderate consumption is safe to include in an anti-inflammatory diet.

Water: Plenty of water! Water is specifically recommended because it can flush toxins and other irritants out of the body. A diet rich in antioxidants and keeping your body hydrated are great ways to reduce inflammation. Natural still water is preferred to carbonated water.

Herbal teas: Teas are great addition to a healthy lifestyle when it comes to warding off inflammation and preventing chronic illness. There are a variety of teas with beneficial anti-inflammatory properties. Ginger, turmeric, and green teas are the most effective to fight inflammations. However, Chamomile, rose petal, black tea, white teas, rooibos, mint, and peppermint are good alternatives.

Lemon juice: It can help reduce swelling and help your body to repair any damaged tissue, thanks to the amount of powerful anti-inflammatory agents contained in lemons.

Clear broths: They are rich in amino acids with strong anti-inflammatory effects. Drinking clear broth straight up is super detoxifying as you put so many good nourishing ingredients inside your body that it literally is forcing the bad stuff out.

NUTS AND SEEDS :

Nuts: Almonds, walnuts, macadamias, and pecans are the nuts with the lowest level of carbs. You should carefully monitor their intake of pistachios, cashews, and chestnuts because they contain a higher amount of carbs. Nuts are best soaked before roasted.

The best low-carb seeds to add to an anti-inflammatory diet are chia and flax seeds which are both full of fiber and omega-3 fats. Sesame seeds are also packed with anti-inflammatory antioxidants, while sunflower seeds contain vitamin E, flavonoids, and other plant compounds that can reduce inflammation.

SWEETENERS :

Stevia: It has the ability to break down the growth and reproduction of harmful bacteria and prevent other infections.

Xylitol: This is an excellent choice with health benefits for your mouth and digestive system. It does not spike blood sugar or insulin.

Keto sweeteners that are allowed in moderation are

Splendor-liquid, Inulin and Chicory root, Lo Han Guo (the monk sweetener with zero calories, zero carbs, zero sugars), and Swerve.

SEAWEED :

Seaweed is low in carbs and is a rich source of a variety of vitamins such as vitamin C, A, E, and B12. It also offers powerful antioxidant, antiviral, and anticancer properties. The consumption of seaweed also helps with weight loss thanks to a low-calorie and high-fiber content, which contributes to increasing the metabolism.
Although most of its calories are from carbs, kimchi is relatively low in them, which means that you can consume it without knocking yourself out of ketosis.

CHOCOLATE :

Dark chocolate contains 50-80% of cacao which is packed with antioxidants that reduce inflammation and provides many health benefits from mood-lifting, improving blood flow, decreasing pain to reducing swelling.

Dark chocolate (at least 75%) is a sweet keto ingredient that can happily be added to your anti-inflammatory diet.

BREAKFAST & BRUNCH

1. CHLORELLA GREEN BOWL

Yields: 2 Servings

Time: 10 mins

Ingredients:

- 2 medium avocados,
- ripe 1 cup cucumber, sliced
- 1 ½ cup almonds milk,
- unsweetened 2 cup spinach
- 2 tsp. chlorella
- powder 2 Tbsp. chia seed
- 1 cup berries, mixed
- ¼ cup raw almonds, chopped

Directions:

1. Blend all the ingredients together until you get a thick creamy texture.
2. Serve with mixed berries and chopped almonds.

Nutrition Fact:

Calories: 445; Fat 33.4g; Cholesterol 0mg; Sodium 171mg; Carbohydrate 30g; Fiber 16.1g; Sugar 7.1g; Protein 12.3g.

2. BASIL-OLIVE EGGS

Yields: 2 Servings

Time: 15 mins

Ingredients:

- 3 large eggs, halved boiled
- 6 kalamata olives, pitted and
- chopped 8 basil leaves, chopped
- 1 Tbsp. extra-virgin olive oil

Directions:

1. Remove the yolk from the eggs and mash it with a fork.
2. Mix the mashed yolks with the basil, olives, and oil.
3. Scoop the mixture into the whites.
4. Refrigerate for 15 mins before serving.

Nutrition Fact:

Calories: 161; Fat 14.6g; Cholesterol 0mg; Sodium 470mg; Carbohydrate 3.5g; Fiber 0g; Sugar 0g; Protein 5.5g.

3. CRISPY BEEF HASH

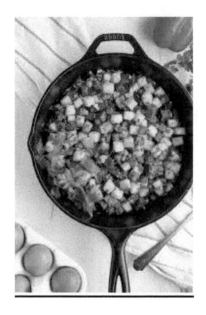

Yields: 2 Servings

Time: 45 mins

Ingredients:

- 1 Tbsp. extra-virgin
- olive oil 2 shallots, diced
- 1 cup radish, diced
- ½ tsp. fresh
- oregano 1garlic clove, minced 1
- ½ cup beef,
- minced
- Seasoning

Directions:

1. Heat the olive oil in a medium frying pan; add shallots, garlic, radish, and seasoning.
2. Sauté for about 5 mins, add the beef and oregano.
3. Mix well and cook for 10 mins.
4. Turn up to the highest heat and press the mixture into the pan's bottom for 2 to 3 mins until the bottom layer gets crispy.

Nutrition Fact:

Calories: 198; Fat 12.5g; Cholesterol 58mg; Sodium 68mg; Carbohydrate 4.4g; Fiber 1.2g; Sugar 1.2g; Protein 21.5g.

4. BREAKFAST ASPARAGUS

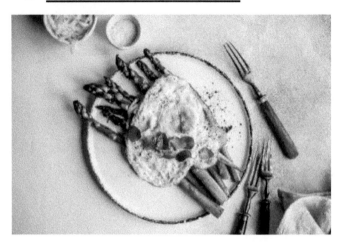

Yields: 2 Servings

Time: 15 mins

Ingredients:

- 4 slices ham, baked
- 12 asparagus, ends
- discarded 1garlic clove
- 1 Tbsp. extra-virgin
- olive oil 4 eggs
- 1 Tbsp. fresh chives,
- chopped Seasoning

Directions:

1. In a cast-iron, heat the olive oil and fry the garlic for 3 mins over medium heat.
2. Add the asparagus and sauté for 5 to 10 mins, depending on the thickness.

3.   When they are almost ready, turn down the heat, add the ham and crack 2 eggs.
4.   Cook until the whites set, keep the yolks running.
5.   Season to taste and serve with chive on top.

Nutrition Fact:

Calories: 325; Fat 19.1g; Cholesterol 377mg; Sodium 1115mg; Carbohydrate 6.2g; Fiber 1.6g; Sugar 4.1g; Protein 31.1g.

5. GRANOLA BAR

Yields: 16 Bars

Time: 45 mins

Ingredients:

- 1 Egg
- 1 tsp. vanilla
- seeds 2 tsp.

  cinnamon
- ¼ cup warm water
- ½ cup macadamia nuts
- ½ cup pecan nuts
- ¼ cup almonds
- ¼ cup sunflower seeds
- ¼ cup flaxseeds
- ¼ cup pepitas
- ¼ cup coconut flakes,
- unsweetened 2 Tbsp. chia seeds
- 2 Tbsp. Stevia, granulated

Directions:

1. Preheat the oven to 340°F.
2. Soak the chia seeds in warm water for 5 mins.
3. Hand chopped pecan, almonds, and macadamia nuts to make small chunks.
4. Mix the nuts, flaxseeds, pepitas, coconut, and sunflower seeds.
5. Add the egg, Stevia, cinnamon, and vanilla into the thickened

chia seeds.

6. Mix all the ingredients and spread them onto a lined baking tray.

7. Bake for 20 mins.

8. Cut into 16 bars.

9. Place the bars over a larger baking tray and return to the oven for a further 15 mins to crisp up.

10. Remove from the oven and cool after they have thoroughly cooled and store in an airtight container.

11. Store in an airtight container for up to 5 days.

Nutrition Fact:

Calories: 487; Fat 48.2g; Cholesterol 85mg; Sodium 40mg; Carbohydrate 22g; Fiber 12g; Sugar 3.9g; Protein 14.6g.

6. VEGGIE OMELET WITH CHEESE & TURMERIC

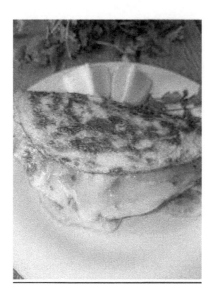

Yields: 2 Servings

Time: 35 mins

Ingredients:

- 3 eggs
- ½ green onion, chopped
- ¼ cup cabbage, shredded
- ¼ red bell peppers, chopped
- ¼ yellow bell peppers, chopped
- ¼ cup fresh cilantro, chopped
- 1 Tbsp. extra-virgin avocado oil
- ¼ tsp. fresh turmeric, grated
- ¼ cup vegetable milk of your choice
- ¼ cup Mozzarella, shredded

Directions:

1. Heat 1 tsp. avocado oil in a pan and sauté the vegetables for 10 mins.
2. Remove from heat and set aside.
3. Into a bowl, beat the eggs with turmeric powder, milk, cilantro, and seasoning.
4. Add the cooked vegetables and mix until well combined.
5. Oil the pan and pour 3 Tbsp. of the beaten mixture, spreading evenly.
6. Sprinkle the mozzarella on top.
7. Cook for 3 mins over medium-low heat until the egg is no longer runny but still gooey. Fold the omelet.

Nutrition Fact:

Calories: 156; Fat 9.7g; Cholesterol 251mg; Sodium 123mg; Carbohydrate 7.5g; Fiber 1.3g; Sugar 3.9g; Protein 11.2g.

BEVERAGES

7. ANTI-INFLAMMATORY LEMONADE

Yields: 2 Servings

Time: 5 mins

Ingredients:

- 1 cup lemon juice, freshly squeezed
- 4–6 cups water
- 1 Tbsp. extra-virgin coconut
- oil 1 tsp. cinnamon, ground
- 1 tsp. fresh ginger, grated
- 1 tsp. fresh turmeric, grated
- ½ tsp. Stevia,
- granulated Pinch sea
  salt

Directions:

1. Place everything in a food processor and blend until thoroughly combined.

Nutrition Fact:

Calories: 175; Fat 5.9 g; Cholesterol 0mg; Sodium 8mg; Carbohydrate 14.8g; Fiber 7.3g; Sugar 5.9g; Protein 3.9g.

8. HIBISCUS MATCHA LATTE

Yields: 2 Servings

Time: 10 mins

Ingredients:

- 2 cup coconut milk, unsweetened
- ¾ cup water
- A handful of dry hibiscus
- flowers 1 tsp. Stevia - optional

Directions:

1. Bring the water to boil, remove it from the heat and infuse with hibiscus flower for 20 mins. Discard the flowers.
2. Warm the milk over low heat, pour in the hibiscus water, and stir well.
3. Add sweetener if you like.
4. Drink hot or shake with ice.

Nutrition Fact:

Calories: 552; Fat 57.2 g; Cholesterol 0mg; Sodium 41mg; Carbohydrate 13.3g; Fiber 5.3g; Sugar 8.1g; Protein 5.5g.

9. ROSEMARY ICED GREEN TEA

Yields: 2 Servings

Time: 10 mins

Ingredients:

- 4 cups water
- 2 lemons
- 4 green tea bags
- 1 Tbsp. Stevia,
- granulated 1 large
  spring rosemary

Directions:

1. Peel the lemons with a vegetable peel, removing all the white bits.
2. In a medium pot, pour in the water, add lemon peels, and Stevia. Stir well to dissolve the sweetener. Bring to boil.
3. Remove from the heat, add tea bags, rosemary and set aside with a lid for at least 30 mins.
4. Remove the tea bags, rosemary, and lemon peels.
5. Squeeze the 2 lemons in, and stir well. Taste and adjust sweetness.
6. Store in the refrigerator to cool.

Nutrition Fact:

Calories: 173; Fat 3.9 g; Cholesterol 0mg; Sodium 8mg; Carbohydrate 12.8g; Fiber 7.3g; Sugar 4.9g; Protein 3.5g.

SOUPS & BROTHS

10. TURMERIC TOFU MISO SOUP

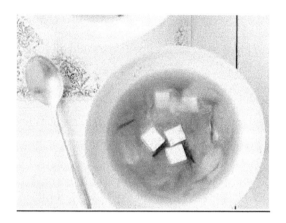

Yields: 2 Servings

Time: 25 mins

Ingredients:

- 1 Tbsp. white mellow miso
- paste 7 oz. tofu, cubed
- 1 tsp.extra-virgin
- avocado oil 7 garlic
- cloves, finely chopped 1
  knob ginger, minced
- ½ red bell pepper, thinly sliced
- ½ head broccoli, chopped
- 2 ½ cups water or more, to preference
- ½ tsp. fresh turmeric,
- grated 1 tsp. apple
  cider vinegar

- 1 tsp. Stevia,
- granulated Scallions
- to garnish Seasoning

Directions:

1. Cook garlic, ginger in a saucepan with avocado oil for about 3-4 mins.
2. Add the peppers and cook for 3 mins more.
3. Add the cubed tofu, broccoli, water, and all the spices (except the miso paste) and bring to a boil.
4. Simmer for 4 mins.
5. Add miso and vinegar, stir well, and simmer for 4 mins.
6. Garnish with scallions and black pepper.

Nutrition Fact:

Calories: 155; Fat 6.2g; Cholesterol 0mg; Sodium 135mg; Carbohydrate 17.1g; Fiber 3.6g; Sugar 4.2g; Protein 11.4g.

11. BROCCOLI & SPINACH SOUP

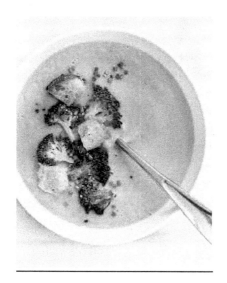

Yields: 2 Servings

Time: 40 mins

Ingredients:

- 1 medium leek
- ½ cup celery, thinly sliced
- 1clove garlic, finely
- chopped 4 cups broccoli florets
- 2 cups water
- 1 tsp. fresh thyme,
- chopped 1 tsp. chives, thinly sliced
- A handful of sunflower
- seeds 1 Tbsp. extra-virgin

olive oil Seasoning

Directions:

1. Rinse the leek and slice it, keeping only the white and light green parts.
2. Heat the oil in a large saucepan over low-medium heat.
3. Add celery and garlic. Fry until they softened.
4. Pour in the water; add all the vegetables, fresh thyme, and seasoning.
5. Bring to boil. Cover and reduce the heat, and simmer until the broccoli are cooked through. Occasionally stir.
6. Let it cool. Transfer to a food processor and blend to get a smooth consistency.
7. Serve warm with sunflower seeds and fresh chive on top.

Nutrition Fact:

Calories: 115; Fat 7.1g; Cholesterol 0mg; Sodium 51mg; Carbohydrate 13.1g; Fiber 3.6g; Sugar 2.9g; Protein 4.4g.

12. WATERMELON GAZPACHO

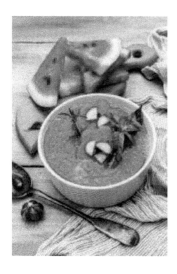

Yields: 2 Servings

Time: 15 mins

Ingredients:

- 1 ¼ cup chunks fresh watermelon
- 2 large roma tomatoes, halved and cored
- ½ small cucumber, peeled and
- seeded 1 small red bell pepper, cored
- 1 small garlic clove,
- peeled 10 fresh mint leaves
- 2 Tbsp. extra-virgin olive
- oil Seasoning
- A pinch of cumin - optional

Directions:

1. Mix all the ingredients in a blender until you get the desired consistency.
2. Taste to adjust seasoning.
3. Store in the refrigerator for 3 to 4 hrs. before serving.

Nutrition Fact:

Calories: 205; Fat 15.1g; Cholesterol 0mg; Sodium 13mg; Carbohydrate 19.8g; Fiber 3.2g; Sugar 13.2g; Protein 3.1g.

13. INSTANT POT SALMON CURRY SOUP

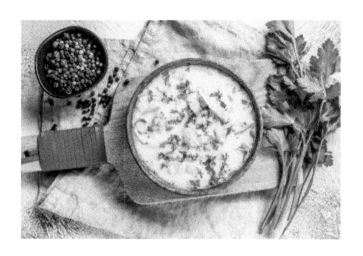

Yields: 2 Servings

Time: 20 mins

Ingredients:

- 2 salmon, skinless
- filets 6 oz. spinach, frozen
- 1 coconut milk, canned
- unsweetened 1 Tbsp. curry powder
- ½ Tbsp. paprika,
- smoked 1 tsp. cumin, ground
- ½ tsp. fresh ginger
- grated $^1/_3$ cup tomatoes,
- stewed Seasoning

Directions:

1. Whisk well the coconut milk with spices and put it into an Instant Pot.
2. Add the frozen spinach and the salmon filets.
3. Cook on Manual, High Pressure, for 15 mins.
4. Quick-release the Instant Pot and serve.

Nutrition Fact:

Calories: 522; Fat 39.1g; Cholesterol 21mg; Sodium 341mg; Carbohydrate 31.5g; Fiber 8.2g; Sugar 6.2g; Protein 18.1g.

14. PEAR, RED PEPPER & TURMERIC SOUP

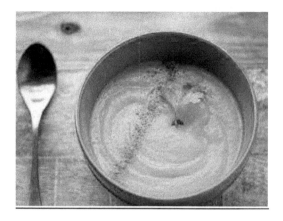

Yields: 2 Servings

Time: 1 hr.

Ingredients:

- 2 small red bell
- peppers 1 shallot
- 1 Anjou pears, peeled and sliced

- 2 cups vegetable broth – see my recipe

- ½ knob fresh turmeric
- 3 Tbsp. extra-virgin olive
- oil 1 Tbsp. fresh chives,
- chopped 2 Tbsp. Greek
- yogurt Seasoning

Directions:

1. Heat 2 Tbsp. olive oil in a medium saucepan.
2. Add the shallots and turmeric, fry over low to medium heat to soften.
3. Add the red pepper and pear and cook for about 8 mins.
4. Pour in the broth, turn to high heat, and bring to boil.
5. Turn down the heat, put the lid, and simmer for 30 mins.
6. Let it cool for 15 mins before transferring it into a food processor.
7. Pulse to obtain a smooth texture.
8. Serve with Greek yogurt and fresh chive.

Nutrition Fact:

Calories: 346; Fat 24.1g; Cholesterol 2mg; Sodium 656mg; Carbohydrate 29.5g; Fiber 6.2g; Sugar 16g; Protein 9.3g.

SALADS & VEGETABLES

15. EGGPLANT PIZZAS

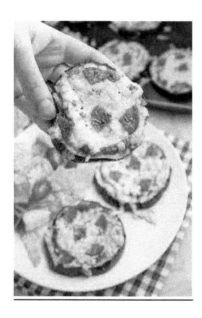

Yields: 2 Servings

Time: 55 mins

Ingredients:

- 1 lb. eggplant, cut into ½ -inch-thick slices, skin
- on 2 Tbsp. extra-virgin olive oil
- 1 cup fresh mushrooms, sliced
- ⅓ cup marinara sauce, reduced-
- sodium 1 cup mozzarella cheese,
- shredded Seasoning

Directions:

1. Preheat the oven to 375°F.
2. Place the eggplant on a paper-towel-lined tray, sprinkle over some salt and let stand for 20 mins.
3. Remove excess moisture using a paper towel.
4. Brush both sides with oil and seasoning; place in on a parchment- paper-lined rimmed baking sheet.
5. Bake for about 15 mins.
6. Increase the temperature and broil.
7. Meanwhile, cook the mushrooms in a pan with 1 Tbsp. oil.
8. Spread marinara sauce evenly over the eggplant slices (2 tsp. each).
9. Place some mushrooms on top and sprinkle evenly with cheese.
10. Broil until the cheese is melted and browned.

Nutrition Fact:

Calories: 247; Fat 18g; Cholesterol 9mg; Sodium 133mg; Carbohydrate 15.2g; Fiber 8.6g; Sugar 7.9g; Protein 7.5g.

16. PORTOBELLO STEAK WITH SPINACH & CHIMICHURRI

Yields: 2 Servings

Time: 40 mins

Ingredients:

- 4 Portobello mushrooms, cleaned and steamed
- removed 3 Tbsp. extra-virgin olive oil
- ½ cup spinach
- 1 garlic clove, minced

- 2 Tbsp. chimichurri
- Seasoning

Directions:

1. Preheat the grill for 20 to 30 mins at the highest temperature.
2. Coat the mushroom with oil and seasoning and place on a baking tray, layer with a piece of parchment paper. Place them on the grill and cook for 5 mins on each side.
3. In the meantime, heat 2 Tbsp. olive oil in a medium pan and cook the garlic for 1 minute over medium heat. Add the spinach to the wilt. Set aside.
4. Plate the mushrooms topped with wilted spinach and a drizzle of chimichurri.

Nutrition Fact:

Calories: 397; Fat 35g; Cholesterol 0mg; Sodium 79mg; Carbohydrate 8.1g; Fiber 1.6g; Sugar 3g; Protein 5.5g.

17. SPINACH & FETA FRITTATA

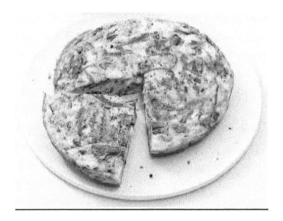

Yields: 2 Servings

Time: 15 mins

Ingredients:

- ½ tsp. extra-virgin olive oil
- ½ cup scallion, sliced
- ½ tsp. garlic, minced
- ⅓ lb. baby
- spinach 2 eggs
- ½ cup feta cheese, crumbled

Directions:

1. Preheat your grill to medium-high heat.
2. Using a non-stick frying pan that you can put under the grill, heat the oil over medium heat.
3. Add the scallion and cook until softened.

4.   Add and Wilt the spinach and toss for a minute.

5.   In a large bowl, beat the eggs, add seasoning, spinach, onion, and feta.

6.   Pour the mixture into the pan over medium heat.

7.   Stir the egg, start gently to set on the bottom.

8.   Place your frying pan under the grill until the frittata is golden and cooked all the way through.

Nutrition Fact:

Calories: 202; Fat 14.1g; Cholesterol 198mg; Sodium 544mg; Carbohydrate 6.7g; Fiber 2.3g; Sugar 2.9g; Protein 15.5g.

18. CAULIFLOWER PIZZA DOUGH

Yields: 2 Servings

Time: 1 hr.

Ingredients:

- 1 ½ lbs. medium-large head of
- cauliflower 1 large egg
- ½ tsp. oregano, dried
- ½ tsp. basil, dried
- ½ cup mozzarella cheese, shredded

Directions:

1. Preheat the oven to 375°F.
2. Line baking sheet with parchment paper.
3. Rinse the cauliflower, remove the outer leaves, separate into florets.
4. Process it in a food processor until "rice" texture forms.
5. Place your cauliflower rice on a prepared baking sheet and bake for 15 mins.
6. Transfer to a bowl and set aside for 10-15 mins.
7. Increase oven temperature to 450°F.
8. In a medium bowl, whisk the egg, dried herbs, and seasoning.
9. Add the cauliflower, Mozzarella cheese, and mix well with a spatula until combined.
10. Line a baking sheet and spray with cooking spray.
11. Transfer cauliflower pizza dough in the middle and flatten with your hands to form the crust.

12. Bake for 20 mins, carefully flip with a spatula, and bake for another 5 mins.

13. Top the cauliflower pizza base with your favorite toppings and bake it again until the cheese is melted.

Nutrition Fact:

Calories: 148; Fat 4.1g; Cholesterol 98mg; Sodium 184mg; Carbohydrate 18.7g; Fiber 9.3g; Sugar 8.3g; Protein 12.5g.

19. GREEK SLAW

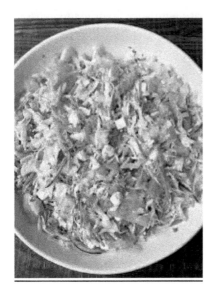

Yields: 2 Servings

Time: 15 mins

Ingredients:

- ½ medium savoy cabbage, finely sliced
- ½ scallion, chopped
- ½ red pepper, chopped finely
- ½ bunch coriander, chopped
- 1 tsp. red chili, finely chopped
- ½ tsp. garlic, minced
- 1 Tbsp. extra-virgin olive oil
- 1 Tbsp. tzatziki – see my recipe
- ½ tsp. Dijon mustard
- ½ tsp. cumin,
- ground Juice of

- lime Seasoning

Directions:

1. Add the tzatziki, mustard, cumin, garlic, seasoning, and lime juice to a large mixing bowl and whisk well until fully combined.
2. Add all chopped vegetables, mix and stir well.
3. Refrigerate for at least 1 hour before serving, sprinkling with chili and coriander.

Nutrition Fact:

Calories: 145; Fat 8.1g; Cholesterol 0mg; Sodium 64mg; Carbohydrate 17.7g; Fiber 7.3g; Sugar 8.8g; Protein 4.5g.

20. TANDOORI GRILLED TOFU WITH RED PEPPERS & BROCCOLI

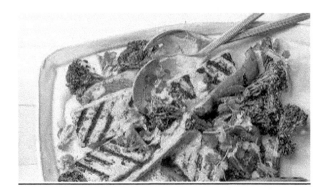

Yields: 2 Servings

Time: 15 mins

Ingredients:

- 1 Tbsp. extra-virgin olive
- oil 1 tsp. chili powder
- ½ tsp. garam masala
- ½ tsp. turmeric, ground
- ½ garlic clove, minced
- ½ tsp. fresh ginger, minced
- ¾ cup whole-milk plain
- yogurt 1 Tbsp. lime juice
- ½ bunch broccoli, trimmed
- ½ medium red bell pepper, sliced
- 8 oz. extra-firm tofu, cut into 2 slices and patted
- dry Fresh cilantro
- Seasoning

Directions:

1. Preheat the grill to medium-high.
2. Heat the oil in a small pan over medium heat.
3. Toast the chili powder, garam masala, turmeric, garlic, and ginger until fragrant.
4. Transfer to a medium bowl, add broccoli, bell pepper, tofu, and coat with yogurt, season with salt and pepper.
5. Oil the grill rack. Grill the tofu, broccoli, and bell pepper, flipping once halfway through, until slightly charred, 6 to 10 mins.

Nutrition Fact:

Calories: 265; Fat 16.1g; Cholesterol 6mg; Sodium 106mg; Carbohydrate 15.7g; Fiber 3.3g; Sugar 9.8g; Protein 18.5g.

21. ROASTED BROCCOLI WITH LEMON-GARLIC VINAIGRETTE

Yields: 2 Servings

Time: 35 mins

Ingredients:

- 1 small broccoli crowns
- 2 Tbsp. extra-virgin olive oil
- ½ tsp. lemon zest
- ½ Tbsp. lemon juice
- ½ garlic clove,
- minced Seasoning to taste

Directions:

1. Preheat the oven to 425°F.
2. Slice broccoli crowns in half. Toss with 2 Tbsp. oil and ¼ tsp. salt in a large bowl.
3. Place them onto a baking sheet and roast until the stems are tender and browned.
4. Meanwhile, prepare the vinaigrette with lemon zest, lemon juice, garlic, pepper salt, and oil.
5. Drizzle the vinaigrette over the roasted broccoli.

Nutrition Fact:

Calories: 145; Fat 14.2g; Cholesterol 0mg; Sodium 17mg; Carbohydrate 3.8g; Fiber 1.4g; Sugar 1.1g; Protein 1.5g.

SEAFOOD DISHES

22. BAKED COD CAKES

Yields: 6 Cakes

Time: 25 mins

Ingredients:

- 8 oz. cod
- 2 eggs
- ¾ cup almond
- flour 2 Tbsp, coconut flour
- ½ tsp. garlic, minced
- ¼ tsp. cumin
- 5 basil leaves,
- chopped 2 thyme
- sprigs Seasoning

Directions:

1. Preheat the oven to 350°F.
2. Line a baking tray with parchment paper.
3. Wash and remove the skin from the cod, cut in small pieces (flakes size).
4. Whisk your eggs in a small bowl.
5. Next, place your cod, flours, spices, herbs, and garlic in a bowl. Add the eggs and mix to combine.

59

6. Roll your mixture into small balls, place them onto the prepared baking tray, and flatten them with the back of a spoon.

7. Press cakes flat with a spoon. The cakes should be about 3 inches wide or so.

8. Bake in the oven for 15–20 mins, until golden brown.

9. Remove and let cool.

10. Season with extra garlic, salt, pepper, if desired.

11. Serve with Greek yogurt.

Nutrition Fact:

Calories: 310; Fat 12g; Cholesterol 226mg; Sodium 155mg; Carbohydrate 13.6g; Fiber 7.6g; Sugar 0.4g; Protein 35.9g.

23. <u>KETO TERIYAKI SALMON WITH STEAMED VEGETABLES</u>

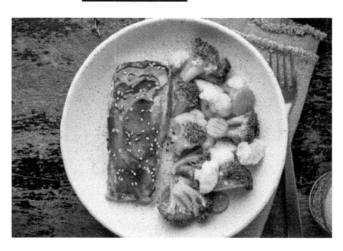

Yields: 2 Servings

Time: 1 hr. 20 mins

Ingredients:

- 1 lb. salmon fillets, cut in
- half 2 garlic cloves, minced
- 1 Tbsp. fresh ginger, minced
- ¼ cup coconut aminos
- 1 cup steamed
- vegetables 1 tsp.
  sesame oil
- 2 tsp. sesame seeds

Directions:

1. Cut your salmon fillet into 2 chunks, marinate with the coconut aminos, sesame oil, garlic, and ginger. Rest in the fridge for at least 1 hour.
2. Toast the sesame seeds and set them aside.
3. Heat a non-stick frying pan over medium-high heat and cook the salmon on each side for about 3–5 mins. (Save the marinade for later.)
4. Once the salmon is cooked, cover it with aluminum foil and set it aside.
5. Add a ¼ cup of water to the leftover marinade and stir to combine.
6. In the same frying pan, add the marinade and bring it to a boil until it thickens.
7. Brush the salmon with the glaze, serve with steamed broccoli and sprinkle over with sesame seeds.

Nutrition Fact:

Calories: 364; Fat 18.9g; Cholesterol 100mg; Sodium 124mg; Carbohydrate 6.2g; Fiber 0.9g; Sugar 0.2g; Protein 46g.

24. SALMON-STUFFED AVOCADOS

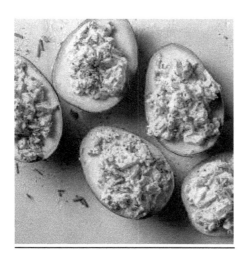

Yields: 2 Servings

Time: 15 mins

Ingredients:

- 5 oz. salmon, skin-off deboned
- ½ cup plain Greek yogurt
- ½ cup celery, diced
- 2 Tbsp. fresh parsley,
- chopped 1 Tbsp. lime juice
- 2 avocados
- 1 tsp. fresh chopped
- chives Seasoning

Directions:

1.   Steam the salmon until cook through.

2. Let it cool for about 15 mins before flaking it.

3. Combine salmon, yogurt, celery, parsley, lime juice, mustard, and seasoning in a medium bowl.

4. Halve avocados lengthwise and remove pits.

5. Scoop about 1 Tbsp. flesh from each avocado half and add to the bowl.

6. Fill each avocado half with the salmon mixture.

7. Garnish with chives.

Nutrition Fact:

Calories: 551; Fat 44.4g; Cholesterol 36mg; Sodium 91mg; Carbohydrate 20.8g; Fiber 14g; Sugar 3.2g; Protein 23.6g.

25. KALE & SHRIMPS SALAD

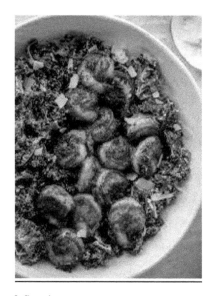

Yields: 2 Servings

Time: 20 mins

Ingredients:

* 8–10 medium-size shrimps, unshelled and
* deveined 2 cups kale, chopped
* 1 Tbsp. extra-virgin olive
* oil 2 garlic cloves, minced
* 1 celery stalk, diced
* ¼ green onion, sliced
* ½ cup fresh
* blueberries 10 fresh

    basil leaves
* 2 Tbsp. coconut milk 1
* tsp. lemon juice

- 1 tsp. extra-virgin olive
- oil Seasoning

Directions:

1. Give the kale a balance, then place in iced water.
2. Heat the olive oil in a frying pan. When hot, add the garlic and stir for 30 secs.
3. Add the shrimps, season, and stir fry for 1 minute. Cover with a lid and simmer the shrimps for 2 mins.
4. Blend all the dressing, dressing ingredients into a food processor until you get a smooth cream.
5. Drain the kale, add the rest of the salad ingredients, and the cooked shrimps into the bowl.
6. Pour some dressing on top and serve.

Nutrition Fact:

Calories: 347; Fat 19.6g; Cholesterol 232mg; Sodium 310mg; Carbohydrate 16.8g; Fiber 2.5g; Sugar 4.3g; Protein 28.6g.

26. CRAB SALAD

Yields: 2 Servings

Time: 15 mins

Ingredients:

- ½ lb. lump crab meat
- 1 romaine lettuce heart, cut
- lengthwise 3 hard-boiled eggs, cut into wedges
- 1 tomato, chopped
- 1 large avocado, diced
- ½ cup plain Greek
- yogurt 1 Tbsp. lemon juice
- 1 tsp.
- paprika
- Seasoning

Directions:

1. Arrange a lettuce bed on two salad plates and top with crab, egg, tomato, and avocado.
2. In a small bowl, combine all the ingredients for the dressing, then drizzle over salads.

Nutrition Fact:

Calories: 487; Fat 30.1g; Cholesterol 345mg; Sodium 859mg; Carbohydrate 20.3g; Fiber 8.6g; Sugar 5.9g; Protein 32.6g.

27. SHRIMPS CAULIFLOWER FRIED RICE

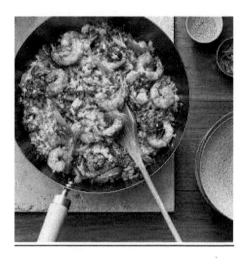

Yields: 2 Servings

Time: 20 mins

Ingredients:

- ¼ cup sesame oil
- 2 large eggs, beaten
- 3 cups cauliflower, riced
- 1 lb. large shrimps, unshelled and
- deveined 3 cups broccoli, florets
- 1 medium red bell pepper, thinly
- sliced 3 garlic cloves, minced
- 2 Tbsp. water, filtered
- 1 Tbsp. apple cider
- vinegar Seasoning

Directions:

1. Pulse the cauliflower to break it down into rice-sized granules.
2. Heat a large frying pan with a Tbsp. oil.
3. Pour the beaten eggs in and fully cook them on one side, flip and cook on the other side.
4. Set aside and cut into small pieces.
5. Add 2 tsp. oil to the pan, heat over high heat. Add cauliflower in an even layer; cook, undisturbed, until lightly browned, 3 to 4 mins.
6. Add 2 tsp. oil to the pan and add the shrimps; cook until just opaque, about 3 mins.
7. Add extra oil to the pan if needed. Add broccoli, bell pepper, and garlic; cook, occasionally stirring, until lightly charred. Stir in coconut aminos, water, vinegar, and pepper. Bring to a boil; boil for 30 seconds. Remove from the heat.
8. Stir in the reserved eggs.

Nutrition Fact:

Calories: 597; Fat 32.1g; Cholesterol 488mg; Sodium 438mg; Carbohydrate 27.3g; Fiber 8.2g; Sugar 9.3g; Protein 55.8g.

28. GRILLED SALMON & VEGETABLES

Yields: 2 Servings

Time: 25 mins

Ingredients:

- 1 lb. salmon fillet, cut into 2
- portions 1 medium zucchini, halved
- lengthwise 2 red bell peppers,
- halved and seeded 1 shallot, cut into
  1-inch wedges
- 1 Tbsp. extra-virgin olive oil
- ¼ cup fresh basil, thinly
- sliced 1 lemon, cut into 4
- wedges Seasoning

Directions:

1. Preheat the grill to high.
2. Brush zucchini, peppers, and shallot with oil and sprinkle with ¼ tsp. salt. Add seasoning to the salmon.
3. Place the salmon and vegetables on the grill.
4. Cook the vegetables for about 6 – 8 mins per side.
5. Cook the salmon, without turning, for about 9 mins.
6. When cool enough to handle, roughly chop the vegetables, and toss them together in a large bowl.
7. Remove the skin from the salmon, serve alongside the vegetables.

Nutrition Fact:

Calories: 426; Fat 22.6g; Cholesterol 105mg; Sodium 118mg; Carbohydrate 17.3g; Fiber 3.5g; Sugar 8.4g; Protein 47.8g

MEAT AND POULTRY

29. ARTICHOKES BAKED CHICKEN

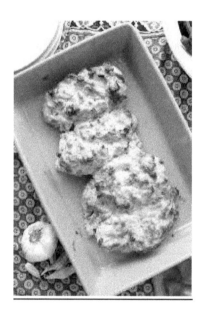

Yields: 2 Servings

Time: 20 mins

Ingredients:

- ½ lb. chicken breast, boneless, skinless 1 ½ Tbsp. extra-virgin olive oil
- ⅓ cup artichoke hearts, sliced
- ¼ cup red chili, finely

- chopped 1 Tbsp. apple cider vinegar
- ½ Tbsp. fresh oregano
- 1 oz. fresh Mozzarella
- cheese Seasoning

Directions:

1. Preheat the broiler to high.
2. In a medium bowl, coat the artichoke hearts with oil, chili, vinegar, and oregano.
3. Heat 1 Tbsp. oil in an ovenproof skillet over medium-high heat and cook the chicken until brown on both sides.
4. Layer the artichoke mixture and cheese on top of each piece of chicken.
5. Place the pan in the oven and broil for 5 to 7 mins until the cheese is melted.
6. Serve with a drizzle of oil and oregano.

Nutrition Fact:

Calories: 378; Fat 21.1g; Cholesterol 118mg; Sodium 213mg; Carbohydrate 7.4g; Fiber 3.6g; Sugar 2.3g; Protein 38.3g.

30. GRILLED CHICKEN WITH GREEK CAULIFLOWER RICE

Yields: 2 Servings

Time: 30 mins

Ingredients:

- 3 Tbsp. + 1 tsp. extra-virgin olive
- oil 2 cups cauliflower rice
- ⅓ cup scallions, chopped
- ½ cup fresh dill, finely chopped
- ½ lb. chicken breasts, boneless, skinless
- ½ tsp. pepper,
- ground 1 ½ Tbsp. lemon juice
- ½ tsp. oregano, dried
- ½ cup cherry tomatoes, halved
- ½ cup cucumber, chopped
- 1 Tbsp. feta cheese,
- crumbled 2 lemon wedges
- for serving Seasoning

Directions:

1. Preheat the grill to medium-high.
2. Make rice-sized cauliflower granules, pulsing the florets in a food processor.
3. Heat 1 Tbsp. oil in a large frying pan over medium heat.
4. Add your cauliflower rice, scallion, ¼ tsp. salt; and cook for

about 5 mins.

5. Stir in ¼ cup dill and remove from the heat.

6. Meanwhile, rub 1 tsp. oil all over the chicken and season with salt and pepper. Grill the chicken for about 15 mins total. Slice crosswise.

7. Serve the cauliflower topped with the chicken, tomatoes, cucumber, olives, and feta.

8. Drizzle with the vinaigrette.

Nutrition Fact:

Calories: 488; Fat 31.3g; Cholesterol 105mg; Sodium 213mg; Carbohydrate 17.4g; Fiber 5.6g; Sugar 5g; Protein 39.3g.

31. CHICKEN, BRUSSELS SPROUTS & MUSHROOM SALAD

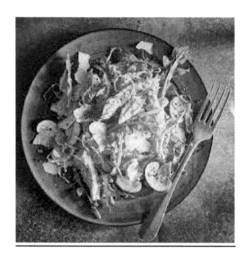

Yields: 2 Servings

Time: 10 mins

Ingredients:

- 6 oz. chicken, shredded and
- cooked 2 cups fresh mushrooms
- 2 cups Brussels
- sprouts 2 cups baby arugula
- ½ cup celery
- 3 Tbsp. extra-virgin olive
- oil 1 ½ Tbsp. apple cider
- vinegar 1 Tbsp. shallot
- ½ Tbsp. Dijon

- mustard 1 tsp.

  fresh thyme
- ½ cup Pecorino
- cheese Seasoning

Directions:

1. Shave the mushrooms and Brussel sprouts, slice the celery, and mince the shallot.
2. Whisk oil, vinegar, shallot, mustard, thyme, and pepper in a large bowl.
3. Add chicken, mushrooms, Brussels sprouts, arugula, and celery; toss to coat.
4. Serve with Pecorino cheese shards.

Nutrition Fact:

Calories: 480; Fat 32.3g; Cholesterol 95mg; Sodium 718mg; Carbohydrate 13.4g; Fiber 5g; Sugar 3.9g; Protein 38.9g.

32. TURKEY COBB SALAD

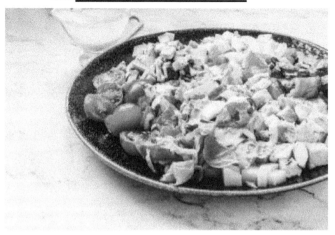

Yields: 2 Servings

Time: 10 mins

Ingredients:

- 1 ½ Tbsp. apple cider
- vinegar 1 ½ Tbsp. extra-
- virgin olive oil 1 tsp. Dijon
  mustard
- 4 cups chopped endive
- lettuce 1 scallion, sliced
- ½ cup cherry tomatoes, halved
- ½ cup cucumber, sliced
- 1 ½ oz. deli turkey,
- cubed 1 hard-boiled
  egg, halved
- ½ cup feta cheese, diced
- ½ avocado, pitted and quartered
- Seasoning

Directions:

1. Whisk vinegar, oil, mustard, salt, and pepper in a small bowl.

2. Place endive, scallions, tomatoes, cucumber, turkey, egg, and feta in a bowl.

3. Just before serving, add avocado, dress the salad, and toss to coat.

Nutrition Fact:

Calories: 380; Fat 30.3g; Cholesterol 126mg; Sodium 819mg; Carbohydrate 12.4g; Fiber 5.9g; Sugar 3.9g; Protein 16.9g.

33. ONE-PAN CABBAGE CHICKEN

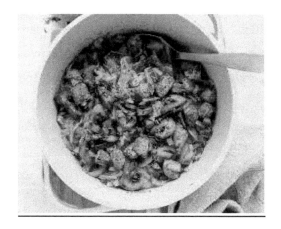

Yields:

Servings

Time: 25 mins

Ingredients:

- 1 lb. chicken thighs
- ½ Tbsp. extra-virgin avocado oil
- ¼ cabbage, finely sliced
- ½ Tbsp. turmeric
- ½ tsp. garlic powder
- 3 green onions,
- chopped 1 ½ cups
  kale
- ¼ cup fresh cilantro, chopped
- Seasoning

Directions:

1. Cut the chicken into small pieces.

2. In a large skillet, cook the chicken to brown over medium heat.

3. In the meantime, hand chops the cabbage and add it to the pan. When the chicken is almost done, add turmeric, garlic powder, and sea salt.

4. Mix to combine, and add the green onions and kale evenly.

5. Stir well and simmer for 3–5 mins.

6. Serve with chopped cilantro on top.

Nutrition Fact:

Calories: 504; Fat 17.3g; Cholesterol 206mg; Sodium 253mg; Carbohydrate 15.4g; Fiber 4.9g; Sugar 4.9g; Protein 69.3g.

34. <u>CHICKEN TACOS IN CABBAGE TORTILLAS</u>

Yields: 2 Servings

Time: 55 mins

Ingredients:

- 1 medium head green
- cabbage 1 lb. chicken
- breasts, boneless 3 Tbsp.
- extra-virgin avocado oil 3
  garlic cloves, minced
- 1 jalapeño, finely
- sliced 2 tsp. cumin,
  ground
- ⅓ cup fresh cilantro,
- chopped 1 scallion, finely
  sliced
- 1 Tbsp. apple cider
- vinegar Seasoning

Directions:

1. Cut the chicken into thin strips. Set aside.
2. In a large pot, bring water to a boil.
3. Discard the outermost leaves of the cabbage.
4. Peel 10 leaves and place them in boiling water for 30 seconds to soften.
5. Dry the cabbage with a paper towel before slicing it into small strips. You should get about 3 cups.

6. Season chicken, cooks it, stirring until browned.

7. Transfer to a plate and add 1 Tbsp. oil and onion to the skillet. Reduce heat to medium and cook, stirring, add garlic, jalapeño, and cumin and cook for about 1 a minute.

8. Stir in the chicken and cover to keep warm.

9. Combine cilantro, scallion, and cabbage in a medium bowl.

10. Whisk vinegar, the remaining 1 Tbsp. oil, and ¼ tsp. salt and stir to combine.

11. Serve the chicken mixture on the cabbage leaves, top with the slaw.

12. Slice the pork and stir any juices into the cherries.

13. Serve together.

Nutrition Fact:

Calories: 257; Fat 11.1g; Cholesterol 98mg; Sodium 113mg; Carbohydrate 5.4g; Fiber 0.6g; Sugar 0.3g; Protein 31.3g.

DIPS, SAUCES & DRESSINGS

35. SARDINE PATE

Yields: 2 Servings

Time: 70 mins

Ingredients:

- ⅓ cup sardines, drained
- ½ Tbsp. fresh capers
- ⅓ cup plain Greek
- yogurt 1 small scallion, sliced
- ½ Tbsp. lemon juice
- ½ tsp. lemon zest
- ½ Tbsp. fresh parsley,
- chopped Seasoning to taste

Directions:

1. Place all the ingredients into a blender and pulse to obtain a smooth consistency.
2. Taste to adjust flavors.
3. Refrigerate for 1 hour before serving.

Nutrition Fact:

Calories: 136; Fat 4.4g; Cholesterol 45mg; Sodium 242mg; Carbohydrate 5.4g; Fiber 0.6g; Sugar 3.9g; Protein 17.9g.

36. <u>CASHEW SOUR CREAM</u>

Yields: 1 cup

Time: 2 hrs. 5 mins

Ingredients:

- 1 cup cashews,
- unsalted 2 tsp. apple cider vinegar
- ½ cup water, filtered
- 2 Tbsp. lemon juice, freshly squeezed
- ½ tsp. nutritional yeast flakes
- ¼ tsp. sea salt

Directions:

1. Soak the cashews for 2 hrs. Rinse and drain.
2. Blend all the ingredients until smooth.
3. Refrigerate in an airtight container for up to 3 days.

Nutrition Fact:

Calories: 430; Fat 32.4g; Cholesterol 0mg; Sodium 256mg; Carbohydrate 27g; Fiber 4.4g; Sugar 3.9g; Protein 15.9g.

37. CREAMY AVOCADO DRESSING

Yields: ½

cup **Time:**

10 mins

Ingredient :

- 1 avocado, peeled and stone
- removed 1 tsp. cumin powder
- 1 large lime,
- juiced 1 Tbsp.
  water
- 1 tsp. lime
- zest 1 pinch
  sea salt
- 1 Tbsp. extra-virgin olive oil

Directions:

1. Blend all the ingredients, except the olive oil, until smooth.
2. Gradually add the olive oil very slowly in a thin stream until the desired creaminess is reached.
3. Refrigerate in an airtight container for up to 3 to 4 days.

Nutrition Fact:

Calories: 93; Fat 9g; Cholesterol 0mg; Sodium 56mg; Carbohydrate 4.3g; Fiber 2.6g; Sugar 0.4g; Protein 0.8g.

38. GINGER & ROSEMARY TAHINI

Yields: ¾

cup **Time:**

10 mins

Ingredient :

- 2 Tbsp. tahini
- ¾ Tbsp. cup fresh lemon juice
- ⅓ Tbsp. Stevia, granulated
- ½ tsp. sea salt
- ½ tsp. ginger, freshly
- grated 2 springs rosemary
- 1 cup water, filtered

Directions:

1. Soak the rosemary in water for at least 30 mins. When the water acquired a rosemary fragrance, discard the rosemary.
2. In a medium mixing bowl, whisk tahini, lemon juice, Stevia, sea salt, and ginger.
3. Gradually add the rosemary until you achieve a pourable.
4. Taste and adjust flavor as needed.
5. Perfect for salads and bowl meals.
6. Refrigerate for up to 1 week.

Nutrition Fact:

Calories: 49; Fat 4.1g; Cholesterol 0mg; Sodium 245mg; Carbohydrate 2.9g; Fiber 0.9g; Sugar 1.1g; Protein 1.4g.

SNACKS

39. <u>SESAME SAVORY CRUNCH</u>

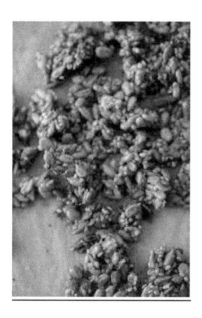

Yields: 2 Servings

Time: 60 mins

Ingredients:

- 1 eggs
- 1¼ cups sesame seeds
- ½ cup sunflower seeds
- 1 Tbsp. psyllium husk powder
- ½ cup
- water

- Seasoning

Directions:

1. Preheat the oven to 350°F.
2. Lay a piece of parchment paper on a baking tray.
3. In a medium bowl, mix all the ingredients, and the mix spread the mixture over the baking tray. Sprinkle with seasoning and bake for 20 mins.
4. Let it cool and cut it into smaller pieces.
5. Put the pieces back into the oven for 30 mins, until lightly golden brown.

Nutrition Fact:

Calories: 558; Fat 46.1g; Cholesterol 164mg; Sodium 75mg; Carbohydrate 23.5g; Fiber 13g; Sugar 0.9g; Protein 20.7g.

DESSERTS AND SMOOTHIES

40. TURMERIC & VANILLA FAT BOMBS

Yields: 6 Fat
Bomb **Time:** 35
mins
Ingredients:

- 1 ½ Tbsp. extra-virgin coconut
- oil 1 Tbsp. grass-fed butter
- 1 tsp. Stevia, granulated
- ½ tsp. fresh turmeric, grated
- ½ tsp. fresh ginger, grated

- ½ Tbsp. almond butter – see my recipe

- ½ tsp. vanilla seeds
- ⅛ tsp. sea salt
- ⅛ tsp. black pepper

Directions:

1. Blend all the ingredients in a blender until smooth and creamy.
2. Select 6 truffle cases and arrange them on a plate. Spoon a Tbsp. the fat bomb mixture into each truffle case.
3. Carefully transfer the plate/molds to the fridge for 30 mins to firm and set.

Nutrition Fact:

Calories: 69; Fat 7.2g; Cholesterol 0mg; Sodium 106mg; Carbohydrate 1.5g; Fiber 0.4g; Sugar 0.4g; Protein 0.7g.

41. GINGERBREAD SUPER BARS

Yields: 8 Bar
Time: 30 mins
Ingredients:

- 1 cup almond flour
- 1 Tbsp. Stevia, granulated
- ½ Tbsp. raw cocoa powder
- ½ Tbsp. ginger, ground
- ½ tsp. cinnamon, ground
- ½ tsp. cloves, ground
- ¼ tsp. baking soda
- ¼ tsp. salt
- ¼ cup grass-fed butter, melted
- ½ large egg
- ¼ tsp. vanilla seeds
- ¼ cup 80% dark chocolate chips

Directions:

1. Preheat the oven to 325°F and grease the metal baking pan.
2. In a large bowl, whisk together the almond flour, Stevia, cocoa powder, ginger, cinnamon, cloves, baking soda, butter, egg, vanilla, and salt until well combined.
3. Then stir in most of the white chocolate chips, reserving a few for topping.
4. Pour the batter into the baking pan, add the chocolate chips to the top.
5. Bake for 20 mins until puffy.
6. Let cool completely before cutting into bars.

Nutrition Fact:

Calories: 77; Fat 6.7g; Cholesterol 12mg; Sodium 146mg; Carbohydrate 4.6g; Fiber 0.6g; Sugar 1.8g; Protein 2.3g.

42. CANTALOUPE CINNAMON CHIA PUDDING

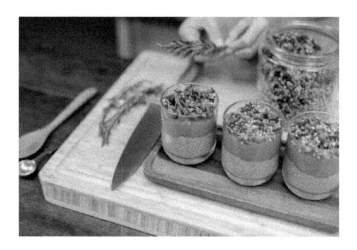

Yields: 2
Servings **Time:**
8hr 10 mins
Ingredients:

- 1 cup almond milk,
- unsweetened 4 Tbsp. chia seeds
- 3 tsp. Stevia, granulated
- ½ tsp. vanilla seeds
- ½ tsp. cinnamon,
- ground 1 cup cantaloupe, diced
- 2 Tbsp. pecans, toasted and chopped

Directions:

1. Stir almond milk, chia, maple syrup, vanilla, and cinnamon together in a small bowl. Cover and refrigerate for at least 8.
2. Mix well, divide into two portions and top both with cantaloupe and pecans before serving.

Nutrition Fact:

Calories: 169; Fat 11.3g; Cholesterol 0mg; Sodium 106mg; Carbohydrate 17.9g; Fiber 7.1g; Sugar 6.5g; Protein 4.3g.

43. CHERRY-SPINACH SMOOTHIE

Yields: 2 Servings
Time: 5 mins
Ingredients:

- 2 cup plain kefir
- 2 cup cherries, fresh or
- frozen 2 tsp. chia seeds
- 1 cup baby spinach leaves
- ½ cup ripe avocado, mashed

- 2 Tbsp. almond butter

- 1 knob ginger, grated

Directions:

1. Place the kefir in a blender. Add cherries; spinach, avocado, almond butter, ginger, and chia seeds, puree until smooth.
2. Serve in a glass.

Nutrition Fact:

Calories: 369; Fat 23g; Cholesterol 0mg; Sodium 64mg; Carbohydrate 34.4g; Fiber 11.8g; Sugar 16g; Protein 11.4g.

44. PEACH AND TURMERIC COCONUT YOGURT

Yields: 2 Servings
Time: 2 hrs.
Ingredients:

- 4 peaches, peeled and sliced
- 1 lb. coconut yogurt, dairy-free
- ½ Tbsp. turmeric, ground, plus extra to serve
- ¼ cup Stevia, granulated
- ½ tsp. vanilla seeds paste

Directions:

1. Blend the peaches in a blender until smooth, then place them in a bowl with all remaining ingredients and whisk to combine.
2. Pour into a shallow container and freeze for at least 2 hrs.
3. Remove from freezer and beat with electric beaters.
4. Return to container and refreeze.
5. Repeat the process until soft-serve consistency.
6. Serve with a little extra turmeric and serve immediately.

Nutrition Fact:

Calories: 194; Fat 2.3g; Cholesterol 0mg; Sodium 28mg; Carbohydrate 44.4g; Fiber 6.5g; Sugar 26g; Protein 3.4g.

BEST ANTI-INFLAMMATORY

45. MACADAMIA

Macadamia is native to Australia, and with 75% fat, it is the fatties nuts ever. The good news is that the majority of it is monounsaturated, and it has an anti-inflammatory effect. Macadamia is also packed with another anti- inflammatory key element, magnesium.

Most nuts are rich in nutrients and beneficial compounds. They are rich in vitamins, fibers, and minerals and help with weight management. Their potential benefits include blood sugar control, overall gut health, digestion improvement, and protection against heart diseases and diabetes.

They have one big downside, though: they are costly. On top of the fact that it takes up to 9 years for the tree to begin producing its fruits and they can be harvest only 5 times a year, the all process is very work- intensely.

MACADAMIA BUTTER

Yields: 1 Jar

Time: 10 mins

Storing: Up to two months in the refrigerator.

Ingredients:

- 16 oz. macadamia nuts
- 6 Tbsp. extra-virgin
- coconut oil 4 Tbsp. Agave
- syrup, optional 1 pinch
  sea salt

Instructions:

1. Blitz the nuts until you get a creamy texture.
2. Add the other ingredients.
3. Blend to get a buttery texture.
4. Place in the refrigerator to set with a shallow layer of coconut oil on top.

Nutrition Fact:

Calories: 354; Fat 35.9g; Cholesterol 0mg; Sodium 28mg; Carbohydrate 11.2g; Fiber 3.6g; Sugar 1.7g; Protein 3.7g.

46. <u>WALNUTS</u>

Walnuts are less expensive than macadamia, a bit higher in carbs (4gr of carbs every ¼ cup) but still considered low in carbs. They are high in Omega- 3 and magnesium, which are an excellent combo for preventing inflammation. Walnuts are perfect for your overall health and ketosis; eating them regularly improves your heart, reduces blood pressure, improves your brain functions, and even helps with weight management.

Sugar-free Candied Walnuts

Yields: 4 Servings

Time: 10 mins

Storing: Up to two months in a sealed container

Note: Cinnamon is not only delicious. Studies have found that it has anti-inflammatory properties as well. It eases swelling and helps to maintain the balance of your stomach, and promotes overall health.

Ingredients:

- 3 cups walnuts
- 1 cup organic coconut sugar
- ¼ cup water
- 1 tsp. vanilla
- seeds 1 tsp. cinnamon
- 1 tsp. sea salt

Instructions:

1. Heat a medium pan over medium heat.
2. Add sugar, water, vanilla seeds, sea salt, and cinnamon. Stir well, frequently.
3. When the sugar completely melted, add the nuts to coat.
4. Remove from the heat and stir again to avoid big clusters.

Nutrition Fact:

Calories: 153; Fat 13.9g; Cholesterol 0mg; Sodium 126mg; Carbohydrate 4.3g; Fiber 1.7g; Sugar 1.7g; Protein 5.7g.

FAVORITES

FAVORITES

THANK
YOU!

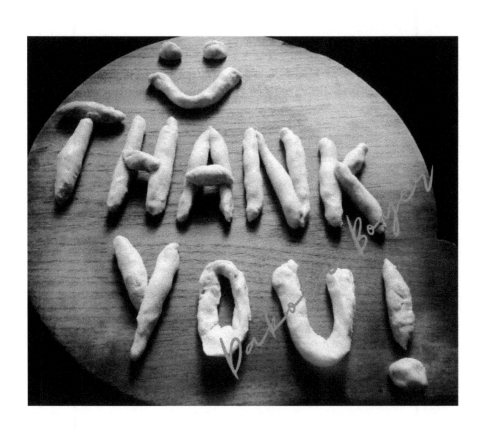

Lightning Source UK Ltd.
Milton Keynes UK
UKHW021845100621
385314UK00002B/273

9 781803 009865